Royal Flush®
The Proof is in the Toilet

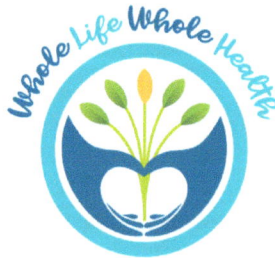

Divine Health is Your Original Design

To the Father of us all:

May we take as much care of our bodies — these "earth suits" — as You did in making them in Your image.

You have provided everything we need to be healthy in spirit, soul and body. Thank You for the journey You've taken us through in our quest for health and well-being. May our lives bring You honor and glory as we follow the path You've laid before us in Your word.

~~~~~~

Our thanks to the health care professionals and others whose input added richly to the body of knowledge contained here.

Our thanks also to the individuals and families who crossed our path looking for solutions with open minds and willing hearts. Their experiences and successes added immeasurably to our journey. We pray that millions more will be blessed!

> *"God put a piece of Himself into every cell of our bodies."*
>
> Barbara Brown

Mere words cannot express the gratitude I have in my heart for Barbara Brown and Dr. Tom Taylor. My life has not been the same since the weekend of March 20-21, 2010, when my 11-year-old daughter and I attended their seminar on health and healing at the invitation of a friend.

My desire to help others gain health and healing began at the age of seven, when my mother was diagnosed with Multiple Sclerosis. By the time I was nine years old, I had decided to become a medical doctor to "cure the world" using western medicine.

Then, when I was 10, I witnessed a miracle: After years in a wheelchair, my mother walked again, while undertaking a simple regimen of mineral baths, massage, exercise, and a special vegetable-based diet in what was then communist Poland. Upon returning home, however, she resumed her usual processed diet, abandoned the

exercises, and was back in her wheelchair within days.

Despite the best medical treatments available, my mother died when I was 16 years old.

Even though I attended Ivy League colleges, medical school, and Family Medicine residency, and had the best training in scientific medicine at the National Institutes of Health, I always knew *something* was missing. I found myself recommending alternative therapies for patients and for my own family, because all too often, people did not get better; they got worse with traditional approaches. The limitations of modern medicine were becoming more and more evident to me.

When my own health crisis came during pregnancy and after the birth of my daughter in 1998, I sought out the best that western medicine had to offer in the "medical Mecca" of Boston, Massachusetts. After 11 years of blood tests, X-rays, and pills, I was left with chronic pain and no answers.

As the old saying goes, *"when the student is ready, the teacher appears."* In my case, two teachers appeared.

I learned more from Barbara Brown and Dr. Tom Taylor in a 2-day workshop about how to restore the mind, body and spirit to true health, than I did in 26 years of schooling and practice!

Could it *really* be this simple, I wondered? Could my daughter and I *really* get better? The answers turned out to be "YES" to both questions.

Of course, the "acid test" came after that weekend seminar. Would I actually invest the time and effort putting into practice what I had learned, or let my busy life and old habits win? But I was desperate, so I committed to perform the cleanses and follow the nutritional recommendations in the book, *Your Personal Road-map to Whole Body Cleansing*, including their *"Essential Non-Negotiable FIVE,"* both of which

may be found at the web site: WWW.WHOLELIFEWHOLEHEALTH.COM.

In addition to the nutritional changes, my daughter and I practiced the **VICTORY MARCH** daily. We also discovered the powerful work of release and forgiveness based on Scriptural principles in the remarkable **HEART, SOUL AND SPIRIT CLEANSE.**

Following the simple action steps in *Your Personal Roadmap to Whole Body Cleansing*, my daughter and I went free from all our former dependencies on prescription and non-prescription medications within the first year. We restored not only our physical health, but our inner sense of peace and well-being in every area of our lives. Most importantly, we found our very *selves* as a result of experiencing truly vibrant health and wellness.

> *"What good is it for a man to gain the whole world, and yet lose or forfeit his very self?"*
> (Luke 9:25, NIV)

My daughter and I continue the habits we established more

than 13 years ago and as a result, we continue to live above pain, illness, or dysfunction, and enjoy our lives fully.

As a Family Physician, I find myself recommending the methods in ***Your Personal Roadmap to Whole Body Cleansing*** more than I pull out my prescription pad. Through my own journey and having the honor of being present with thousands of patients and their families on their journeys, I have found that there is a more excellent way: God's way. It was always there, right under our noses.

I thank the Lord for Barbara Brown and Dr. Tom Taylor, and for their dedication to serving others, no matter the time of day or the difficulty of the situation. They are true healers who share their knowledge generously and with great love.

As you embark on this most amazing journey, I encourage you to read and re-read, and actually ***DO*** what they recommend in this book.

> *"Don't deceive yourselves by only hearing what the word says, but do it."* (James 1:22, CJB)

When you put the wealth in ***Your Personal Roadmap to Whole Body Cleansing*** into action, you will have taken *"the road less traveled,"* as the poet, Robert Frost, so aptly put it, and that *will* make *"all the difference."*

Joy, peace, and blessings
on your unique personal journey.

Claudia G. Gabrielle, MD, FAAFP

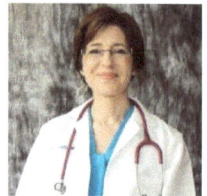

TABLE OF CONTENTS

GUIDING PRINCIPLES

We have found the following principles to be 100 percent reliable:

Spiritual Principles

1. Merging science and scripture is essential to gain clear understanding of how your body works, how you get sick, how you get healthy, and how you stay that way.

2. Scriptural principles are entirely practical, 100 percent reliable, and applicable, whether you believe them or not.

3. You are a spiritual being undergoing a physical experience, not the other way around. When you live like physical beings looking for a spiritual experience, you are 180 degrees out of phase with how God created you.

4. Pain, illness, disease, or dysfunction, is the inevitable result of being out of alignment with God's original blueprint

5. Healing is inevitable and unstoppable when you align and agree with God's divine design.

Physical Principles

1. Your body is self-organizing, self-healing, and self-regulating.

2. Your body does not think, judge or reason.

3. Your body responds for only one purpose: survival, and the response is perfect for the stimulus that makes it necessary.

4. Your body's responses don't always feel good (we call those symptoms), but they are perfect nevertheless.

5. Your body is an alkaline organism by design. It creates acid as a byproduct of being alive, and you add to that acid load by the choices you make in eight key areas (see page 102 in the book, *Your Personal Roadmap to Whole Body Cleansing*).

6. Your physical design (your anatomy) – tooth structure, digestive tract, enzyme production, and absorption process – is suited to a primarily plant-based diet.

7. Your body is constantly cleansing, rebuilding and supporting the life within every cell and between all cells.

Principles like those above hold true no matter what your gender, race, ethnicity, or beliefs. The good news is that you are in charge of the choices that enable your body to perform at peak efficiency, according to its original design. Any level of performance less than that is the natural consequence of your choices in eight key areas we discuss on page 102 of the book, *Your Personal Roadmap to Whole Body Cleansing*.

Finally, your body responds according to its design, not to your desire. You probably know people who genuinely want to be well, yet vibrant health seems to evade them. All our combined experience has proven that when you align yourself with God's design – spiritually, mentally, and physically – illness cannot hold you hostage; instead, health, happiness and success is the inevitable outcome.

Sound good?

Let's get on with it, shall we?

Barbara Brown, MSE
Dr. Tom Taylor

INTRODUCTION

Cleansing, rebuilding, and supporting are normal activities that go on continually in every cell, tissue, organ, and system of the body. At the center of these processes you'll find minerals. Minerals are essential for all life and without them, life ends. When you are deficient in minerals – and you need around 70 – you lose quality of life by degrees. The good news is that the opposite is also true: When you replenish your body's supply of minerals daily, you *gain* quality of life in significant ways:

- **Memory improves** – walk into a room and remember why!
- **Immunity increases** – fight off illness easily!
- **Flexibility and mobility improves** – move easier!
- **Sleep improves** – sleep like a baby, even if you're 90!
- **Weight normalizes** – eliminate stubborn weight and look younger!

Help your body run like a well-oiled machine!

Like our friends, family and clients, we pray that you will also enjoy the benefits above and more!

Blessings and joy on your journey,

Barbara Brown, MSE
Dr. Tom Taylor

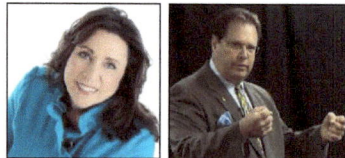

THE ROYAL FLUSH®
A SAFE AND EFFECTIVE DETOXIFYING INTESTINAL CLEANSE

The ROYAL FLUSH®, when used to replace one meal per day, is a superior, safe, easy, and effective method of cleansing years of built-up waste in the entire intestinal tract – *not just the colon* – and ridding the body of accumulated toxins. Many methods of colon cleansing are available and some are more effective than others. They may include pills, capsules, powders, suppositories, candies, chewing gum, drinks, enemas or colonics, and even surgical procedures.

According to experts in the field of natural health, many chronic health problems have their origin in poor dietary habits, faulty digestion, lack of efficient nutrient absorption, and poor elimination of waste.

Elie Metchnikoff, the Nobel prize-winning Russian biologist, is credited with the statement, *"Death begins in the colon,"* which is often evidenced by a host of symptoms, some of which are so slight as to go unnoticed or be taken for granted as part of normal aging processes.

"Leaky Gut Syndrome" is a common diagnosis given to those with symptoms of toxic build-up in the intestines.

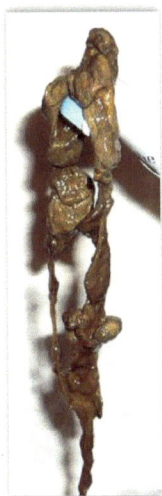

You may find it hard to believe that built-up waste like this picture could be in your intestines, but the proof is in the toilet! If you've eaten white flour, white sugar, fried, processed or fast foods, or have not had proper elimination (2 to 3 times a day), you would benefit from the ROYAL FLUSH®!

Most people enjoy a decrease in food cravings, stabilized appetite, increased energy, improved memory, and elimination of excess fat and weight. They may be preventing other health problems too!

Residue of built-up waste in the intestines may become hardened, creating a "pipe" around the lining of the tissue walls, which prevents efficient assimilation of nutrients needed for optimum health. Venus Andrecht, author of *The Herb Lady's Notebook*, interviewed nurses who assisted surgeries during which colons had to be removed with a hacksaw!

Some people may have malformed colons with kinks, bulges, balloons or collapsed areas and others may also have restrictions due to accidents or surgery. Obstructions can also occur in the small intestines.

All of these areas are potential problems since waste accumulation allows toxins to be released into the blood stream and recycled through the entire body.

Normal bowel movements should occur two to three times per day. If this is not the case, consider performing the simple and effective **SALTWATER FLUSH** on page 8 as a way of encouraging normal bowel movement.

Commercial products to assist bowel movement and regularity, and the amount needed, will vary from individual to individual. If you choose such a preparation, start by using the directions on the label, and increase or decrease the amounts slowly to achieve the desired results.

If you are accustomed to infrequent bowel movements, it may take several weeks to establish proper activity.

Before beginning the ROYAL FLUSH®, be certain your bowels are moving two to three times a day for at least a week.

If this is not the case, the SALTWATER FLUSH on page 8 is an effective way to stimulate the bowels naturally, without resorting to harsh laxatives.

INGREDIENTS FOR THE ROYAL FLUSH®

STEP 1 – DETOX CLAY

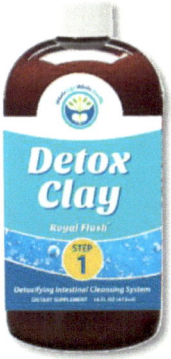

All natural Bentonite works like a magnet to attract toxic substances, clean out mucus, and assist in their rapid removal. **DETOX CLAY** is no longer available, but **SONNE'S #7** is an equally powerful detoxifying agent, absorbing up to 40 times its own weight in toxins, and helping rid the body of harmful bacteria and parasites.

STEP 2 – TRACE MINERALS PLUS+®

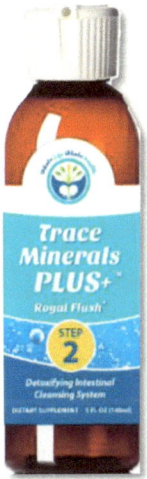

The key to the **ROYAL FLUSH®** is a unique solution of macro minerals and trace elements derived from an ancient plant deposit. Among other benefits, **TRACE MINERALS PLUS+®** is believed to help the body handle toxins, kill parasites, naturally chelate heavy metals, supply essential trace elements missing in foods and most supplements, and generally create an internal environment that resists disease–causing organisms. No other minerals we have tested work as well in the **ROYAL FLUSH®** as **TRACE MINERALS PLUS+®**.

STEP 3 – CLEAN SWEEP MIX™

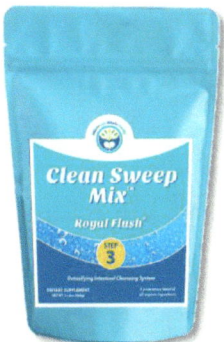

An all-organic, proprietary blend of soluble and insoluble fibers, plus organic super greens. When mixed with apple juice and water, the **CLEAN SWEEP MIX™** works like a broom, cleaning the digestive tract and nourishing it at the same time. **CLEAN SWEEP MIX™** is no longer available, but we've shared the recipe on page 5 so you can DIY at home!

Apple Juice: Organic, unfiltered apple juice contains slower burning, more satisfying carbohydrates than processed apple juice, and provides a great source of energy (fresh, non-pasteurized apple cider is even better). Whole-leaf aloe vera juice may be substituted if allergies, blood sugar problems, or Candida (yeast) prohibit the use of apple juice.

Optional Probiotics: *Acidophilus* and *Bifidus* are examples of healthy bacteria, called Probiotics, which help re-establish a proper intestinal environment as waste and toxins are flushed out. Probiotics should be taken at least 30 minutes before – or hours after – meals or the ROYAL FLUSH® to ensure that the beneficial bacteria are not denatured in the stomach before they reach the intestinal tract.

THE PROOF IS IN THE TOILET!

Many people eliminate parasites while on the ROYAL FLUSH®, in addition to tumors, and unidentifiable masses of varying shapes, colors and sizes. **The proof is in the toilet!**

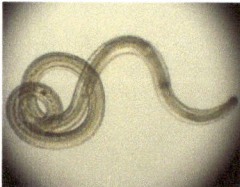

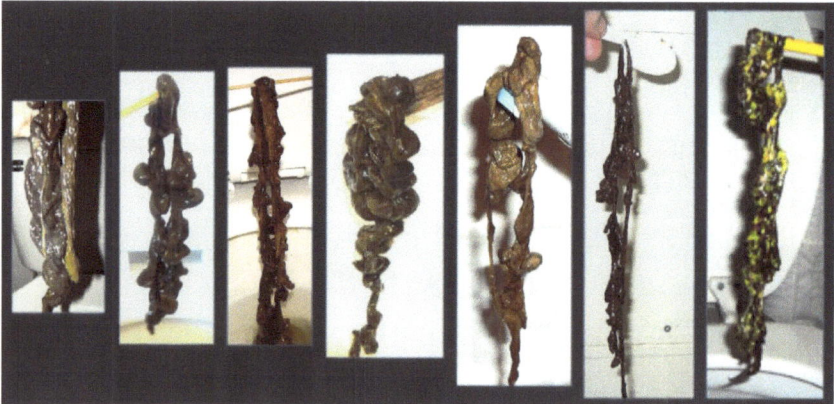

DIY ROYAL FLUSH® RECIPE

FIRST: On an empty stomach, take 1 tablespoon SONNE'S #7

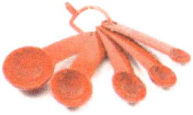

- **3 hours before flush** (2 hours works, but 3 is better).
- **Use a plastic measuring spoon** – never let it touch metal!
- **Rinse your mouth after swallowing**, and sip a little water.

SECOND: Mix in your BlenderBottle® (2-3 hours after Sonne's #7)

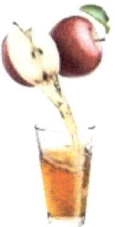

- **12 oz. organic apple juice** *(Use whole leaf aloe vera juice for Candida or blood sugar problems)*
- **12 oz. ALKALINE IONIZED**, reverse osmosis, or filtered water
- **1 teaspoon* TRACE MINERALS PLUS+®**
- **3 level Tablespoons* of CLEAN SWEEP MIX™** – Recipe:
  - **21 oz (600 grams) of organic psyllium husk powder**
  - **7 oz (200 grams) of organic whole psyllium husk**
  - **3.5 oz (100 grams) of organic green power blend**
  - *Use only ½ amounts for the first three to four days.

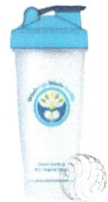

THIRD: Shake well and drink fast! (The fiber in CLEAN SWEEP MIX™ swells quickly.) Wait for 2-3 hours to eat.

Continue the **ROYAL FLUSH®** until all abnormal, rubber-like, hardened, mucus-like toxins are eliminated. Continue for an additional two weeks, then stay off for two weeks, and then try the flush again to see if any more abnormal toxins are eliminated. If not, repeat the **ROYAL FLUSH®** once a week or at least once a month, depending on your diet.

The first **ROYAL FLUSH®** "adventure" may take a few weeks to a few months to complete.

Brush your teeth after drinking the ROYAL FLUSH®, so that TRACE MINERALS PLUS+® won't stain your teeth!

THE PROCESS

Replace one meal every day with the ROYAL FLUSH® (no food for 2-3 hours before, during or after). Replacing breakfast is a popular practice, although some people find it easier to replace lunch or dinner. Whatever meal you choose to replace, it is essential to drink all of the ROYAL FLUSH®. Remember that the "broom" (**CLEAN SWEEP MIX™**) needs volume to "push" it.

It is normal to experience varying degrees of abdominal bloating and distention. Depending on the level of toxicity in your body, mild headaches or slight, flu-like symptoms may occur. Before being completely eliminated, toxins will be released into the blood stream after being loosened from the intestinal walls. To eliminate unpleasant symptoms, use only half the recipe for the first three to four days, and then increase to the full recipe.

Continue the ROYAL FLUSH® until the stool looks normal for at least 7 consecutive days. The duration of this cleanse is determined by the extent of accumulated waste. An adult who has never cleansed his or her colon should plan to be on the ROYAL FLUSH® for at least three months, or until the desired results are reached.

> **The Proof is in the Toilet!**
>
> When you find black, rubbery, hardened, rope-like, mucous-laden material at the end of your TREASURE STICK™, you'll know your intestines are being cleaned out!

Other cleansing regimens that you may want to consider, along with the ROYAL FLUSH®, include the two-week **LIVER REJUVENATING PROGRAM**, followed by the **4-DAY KIDNEY, LIVER AND GALLBLADDER CLEANSE**. These and other cleanses may be found in the book, *Your Personal Roadmap to Whole Body Cleansing*.

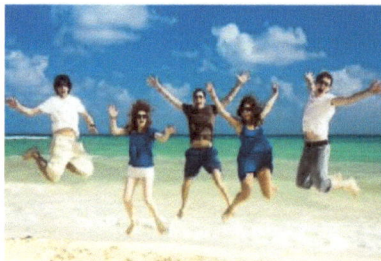

TIPS FOR THE ROYAL FLUSH®

- **The CLEAN SWEEP MIX™ contains super green foods** for added, concentrated nutrition, to restore, build, and support your cells while you're cleansing.

- **The CLEAN SWEEP MIX™ also contains a unique soluble fiber blend** that has proven to be the most effective by far without being harsh.

- **You may need help to eliminate rubbery waste.** An already clogged colon requires an extra "push." See the **SALTWATER FLUSH** on page 8. Work with a holistic practitioner to determine what works best for you. Avoid prescription drugs if possible.

- **There may be bloating and gas during the first three or four days.** To reduce or eliminate burping, gas and bloating, use digestive enzymes with meals and snacks, and/or between meals.

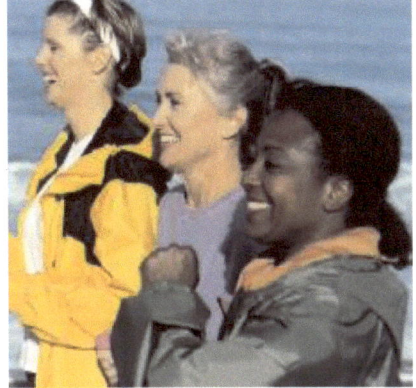

  One of many excellent books to read on the importance of enzymes is *Enzymes – The Missing Link to Vibrant Health*, by Dr. Humbart Santillo.

- **To maintain detoxification**, eat lots of vegetables, and *very little* animal protein.

Our thanks to the late John B. Scott for his work in first developing the Royal Flush® using Trace Minerals Plus+®, and to his daughter, Jan Scott Johnson, for her kind permission to use her late father's material.

THE SALTWATER FLUSH

FOR BOWELS THAT NEED A LITTLE HELP

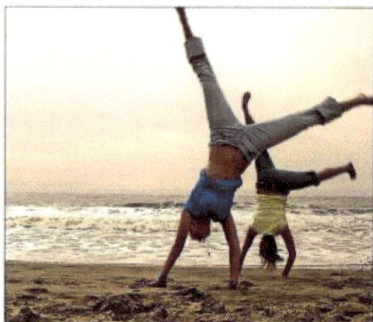

Salt has been used throughout the ages to draw out poisons and as an anti-bacterial agent. The **SALTWATER FLUSH** provides an internal bath, flushing toxins without the harmful effects of chemical laxatives. Unlike colonics or enemas, which can only reach into the large intestine, or a small part of it, the **SALTWATER FLUSH** removes toxins as it cleanses the entire digestive tract from the top down.

Salt will do no harm when used in this way, and will sterilize, making it easier for the body to repair the tissues.

SALTWATER RECIPE

- **2 level teaspoons of unrefined sea salt.** *(Do not use ordinary iodized salt.)*

- **1 quart warm water.**

- **Mix in a 1-quart container.** Shake or stir well to dissolve completely.

- **Drink the entire quart of saltwater first thing in the morning.** It must be taken on an empty stomach. *Using a straw can make it easier to drink the mixture.*

- **Lie on your right side for 30 minutes** after drinking the saltwater.

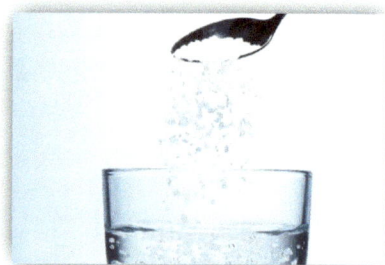

TIPS FOR THE SALTWATER FLUSH

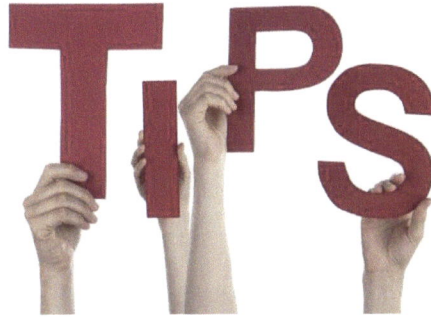

➤ The saltwater mixture will not be absorbed and will stay intact to wash the entire digestive tract thoroughly in just a few hours.

➤ Most people will have bowel elimination in 1 to 2 hours.

   ✓ **Multiple eliminations are common.**

➤ **Be careful passing gas:** Liquid will be coming through your system.

➤ **The SALTWATER FLUSH** can be used daily if needed.

➤ **If constipation has been a chronic problem**, it may be advisable to take an herbal laxative tea, or the herb, *cascara sagrada*, at night to loosen fecal matter and then drink the **SALTWATER FLUSH** the next morning.

WHAT ARE MINERALS AND WHY DO I NEED THEM?

Your body functions according to God's design, not your desire. The natural order works only one way:

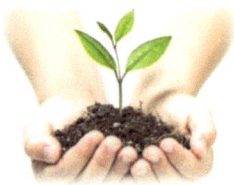

- **The Mineral kingdom feeds the Plant kingdom**
  - **Plants derive minerals from the soil**

- **The Plant kingdom feeds the Animal kingdom**
  - **Animals derive minerals from plant foods**
  - **Animals cannot derive usable minerals directly from the soil**

Minerals are essential nutrients that facilitate more than 10,000 chemical reactions taking place each second at the same time in trillions of cells in your body's tissues, organs...even your bones!

Minerals exist naturally in the soil, but you can't absorb them in this "elemental" or "metallic" form. Humans and animals must derive their minerals from plants, which have broken down material from the soil and rocks into minute, organic particles that are recognizable, absorbable, and usable in your body.

• What do minerals do in my body?

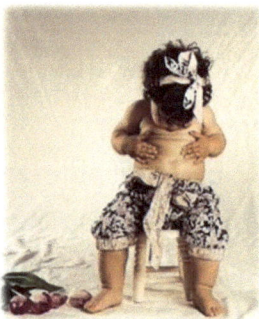

Most of us know that minerals build bones, but minerals are also behind the building up, supporting, cleansing, and tearing down processes that occur every day throughout every organ and tissue. Tens of thousands of enzymes depend on minerals to make chemical reactions occur. Minerals literally make things happen in your body, and without them nothing works.

"In the absence of minerals, vitamins have no function. Lacking vitamins, the system can make use of the minerals, but lacking minerals, vitamins are useless."

Dr. Charles Northern MD. researcher in the 1930s

• What is the difference between minerals and "trace minerals"?

Minerals are categorized as "major elements," or "macro minerals"; "minor elements," and "trace elements" (and recently, "ultra-trace elements") or "trace minerals." Macro minerals are required in relatively large amounts (over 100mg); they include sodium, potassium, magnesium, calcium, phosphorus, and chloride. Minor elements and trace elements are often categorized together as trace minerals. The name comes from the tiny amounts found in nature and required in the body. Many trace minerals measure more than 1,000 times less than macro minerals, and some are barely measurable at all. Zinc, iron, copper, iodine, and manganese, are among the most commonly recognized trace minerals.

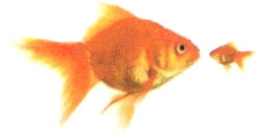

Our soil has been depleted of many minerals since the advent of modern farming in the early 1900s. Even a diet rich in organically grown vegetables and fruit is deficient in minerals that were once plentiful.

• What are some signs of a mineral deficiency?

Dr. Linus Pauling, two-time Nobel prize winning scientist, was quoted as saying, *"You can trace every sickness, every disease, and every ailment to a mineral deficiency."*

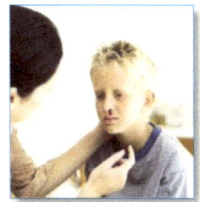

> **Some of the landmarks of mineral deficiency include dry skin, acne, poor reflexes, anemia, apathy, general weakness, confusion, sleeplessness, headaches, depression or anxiety, constipation or diarrhea, confusion or memory loss, shortness of breath, dandruff, hair loss, susceptibility to illness, poor sense of taste or smell, and hormonal imbalance.**

It's easy to see why a mineral supplement has become an important daily requirement for optimal function, disease prevention, and long-term health and well-being.

• Can I get minerals from a daily multivitamin?

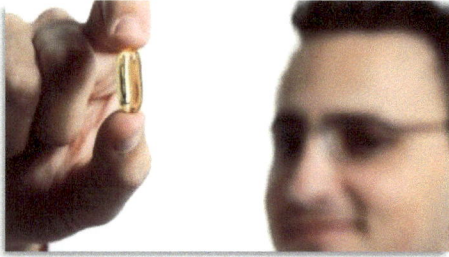

Most vitamin or vitamin/mineral supplements contain only a few of the more than 70 minerals that should be available. Even then, depending on their source and manufacture, only a small amount of any mineral may actually be usable in your body. As one doctor put it, "*Most vitamin/mineral supplements simply become expensive urine.*"

• Are there any scientific studies on minerals?

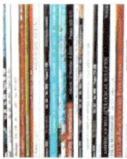

Thousands of scientific studies have been published on the function of specific minerals, their "Recommended Daily Allowance,"* sources, relative safety, signs of deficiencies, and dangers of toxicities.

> ***The RDA has long been recognized as a minimal intake, below which signs of deficiencies are known to occur over time.**

• Why doesn't my doctor recommend or prescribe minerals?

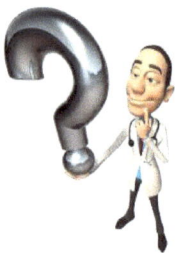

Patients often have more knowledge of nutrition than their doctors. Physicians are trained in pharmacology (drug therapy). Only in that realm are prescriptions permitted legally. Most doctors receive scant training, if any, in the science of nutrition, let alone nutritional supplementation.

Many doctors are aware that "micronutrients," such as vitamins, phytonutrients (nutrients from plants), and minerals, play an important role in human health. Unless your doctor has undertaken extensive study and training in nutrition, he or she is ill-equipped to make dietary or supplement recommendations.

With a few exceptions, medical doctors are not your best sources of knowledge or recommendations regarding nutrition or nutritional supplements.

• What are the differences between mineral supplements?

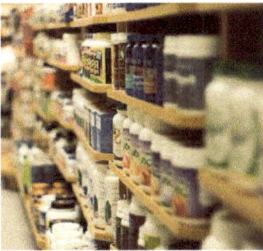

Mineral supplements come in many forms, from chalk (calcium carbonate) to shells or coral; from rocks to salt or plant deposits; many are extracted – or even worse, synthesized – in laboratories. You'll find tablets, capsules and various kinds of liquids.

> **The worst part for consumers is that nearly every mineral supplier claims to have the best source, manufacture, purity, absorbability, and efficacy.**

• So, what is the best way to take minerals?

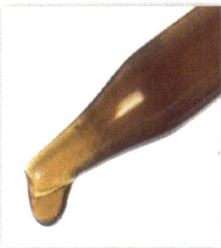

The best mineral "delivery system" we've found is a **liquid**. Tablets, capsules, and even powders, fall short on two counts: First, many contain unnecessary binders or fillers; and second, you'll find that the **full spectrum** of minerals that ought to be available to your body is present only in liquids.

All liquids are not created equal! Beware of products that require ounces per day as a normal amount. You should be able to use up to only a teaspoon per day.

> **Traveling to a country where bacteria or parasites may contaminate the food or water?** You may need to take several teaspoonfuls of liquid minerals per day to avoid dysentery and discourage other parasitic invasions.

• How do I know that minerals are absorbed by my body?

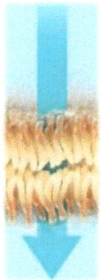

The quickest, simplest, least costly way to know whether you are absorbing the minerals you take is to monitor the signs of mineral deficiency on page 11. Scientists and doctors often dismiss testimonies, or what they call "anecdotal evidence"; costly tests, such as hair analysis, may help "prove" effectiveness; however, our experience is that you know better about how your body feels than any scientist.

• What effects can I expect from taking minerals?

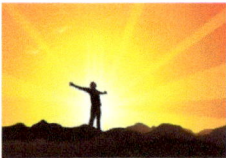

"Expect" is a loaded word, and we can't promise anything from taking liquid minerals. If you're like many we've served over more than two decades, the most obvious signs of improvement include increased energy, improved memory and focus, a higher functioning immune system, and better sleep.

Being deficient in minerals results in a lower quality of life than you deserve, with less resistance to disease, and possibly even a shorter life span. Functioning at the highest level possible in every area of life is impossible to achieve without sufficient minerals. If living at your best and fulfilling the purpose for which you were created is important to you, adding minerals to your daily nutritional regimen is imperative.

• How much of any one mineral should I take?

Drops, NOT ounces!

Most nutrients occur naturally in very small amounts; so, a few drops of the right, full-spectrum, liquid mineral supplement is far better than taking any amount of *one* mineral or group of minerals. The intelligence that God designed in your body will select how much of each nutrient to use at a particular time, so long as you provide *all* the known major, minor and trace elements, in a form your body can *recognize*, *absorb*, and *utilize*.

Studies show that nutrients work best in their natural state, surrounded by other nutrients that work together. For example, we know that calcium, magnesium, phosphorus, and even Vitamin D, are all absorbed and function better when they are all present at the same time, even if the amounts of any one of those minerals is very small.

> **The right amount of any one mineral is exactly what your body requires at any given time. The only way to know is to avoid man-made formulas and rely on what God originally created in nature to work together with everything else He created.**

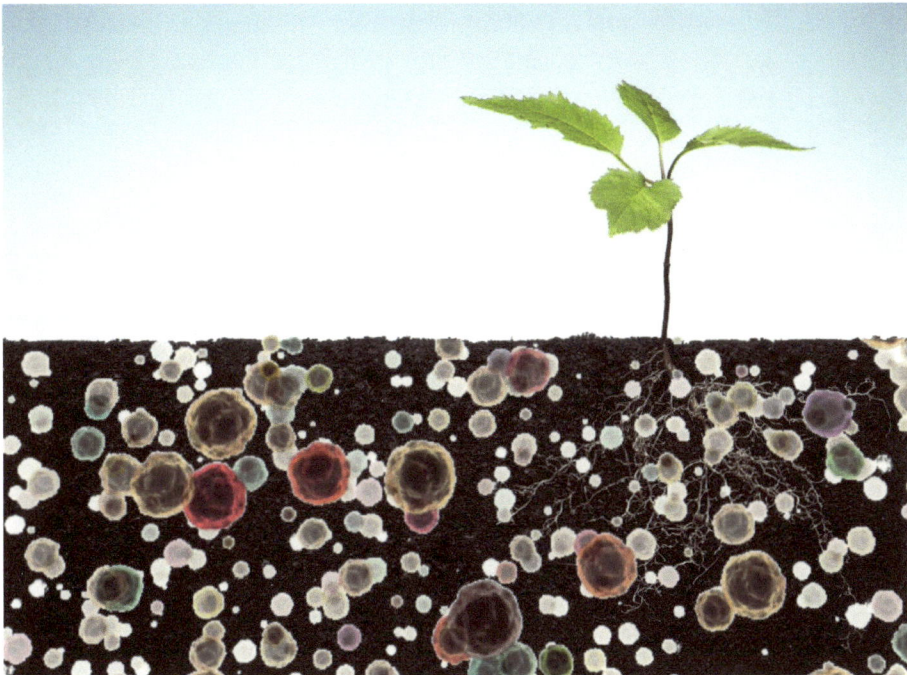

WHAT ARE THE BEST SOURCES OF MINERALS?

The best mineral supplements come from ancient plant deposits. Tens of millions of years ago, before anyone farmed anything, the full spectrum of more than 70 minerals was available in the soil. The minerals were taken up by the plants that grew abundantly at the time; as those plants died and decomposed, they naturally replenished the soil with the same minerals. The cycle was repeated over millions of years until an enormous amount of naturally organic material was built up, called *"humic shale"* or *"humic clay."*

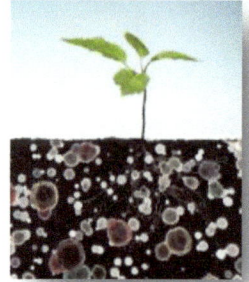

> **Two Amazing Facts**
>
> **Minerals from soil, rocks, salts, or shells – anything other than plants – are in an *"elemental"* or *"metallic"* state, and are therefore useless to your body.**
>
> **Plants miraculously change unusable minerals into a form your body can recognize, absorb and utilize for every task – every cellular reaction – exactly as God intended.**

• How do minerals become liquid?

Today, we can tap an ancient, composted plant deposit – which looks like coal – dry it until it becomes a sandy consistency, drip water through it – s l o w l y – and produce a liquid, called a *"colloid."* This amber-colored liquid appears to be a clear solution, but it contains millions of microscopic mineral particles, so small that they are always suspended in the water.

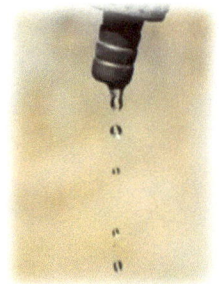

- ## The miracle of "Fulvic Acid"

TRACE MINERALS PLUS+® also contains *"fulvic acid,"* a naturally occurring organic substance that is created by microbial action between ancient, mineral-rich soils and prehistoric plant deposits that have composted over millions of years. Fulvic acid is highly bioactive and is believed to enable nutrient absorption in plants, and then transforms those nutrients into complexes that you can absorb.

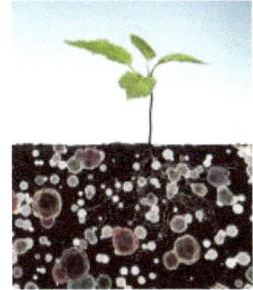

Fulvic acid is found in rare plant deposits, sometimes called humic clay. Although it is not clearly understood, or overlooked, by most of the scientific and medical community, fulvic acid's unique characteristics, gives TRACE MINERALS PLUS+® a kind of *"living"* property.

Some of the actions that fulvic acid seems to demonstrate:

- Increased energy
- Improved immunity
- Heavy metal elimination
- Wound disinfection, treatment
- Free radical scavenging
- Restored electrolyte balance
- Increased enzyme activity
- Improved blood pressure

- ## Do liquid minerals contain all the nutrients I need?

The subject of how many nutrients are required by human beings is controversial and hotly debated in scientific circles even in the 21st century. Amazingly, as late as the mid 1980's, scientists added nutrients such as chromium, nickel, tin, vanadium, and boron, to a list of only 15 minerals considered as essential or beneficial. The exact benefits of at least 55 other minerals are still unknown or unstudied.

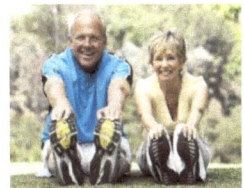

> **Before anyone farmed anything, more than 70 minerals were present to support human life!**

Liquid minerals, from the right source, can provide all the minerals that are needed in small amounts; other food sources are required for minerals that you need in much greater amounts.

> Liquid minerals do *NOT* supply *ALL* the nutrients you need – they supply nutrients you absolutely *MUST* have and *WON'T* find anywhere else!

• What mineral supplement do WE use every day?

TRACE MINERALS PLUS+® comes from people we know and trust, whose family pioneered much of the earliest work on minerals in the early to mid 1900s, for both agricultural use and human consumption. The intestinal cleanse, known as the ROYAL FLUSH®, was originally developed by the patriarch of this family, who recognized the uncommon healing properties of TRACE MINERALS PLUS+®. The family has kept pure the prehistoric plant deposit, which is the source of TRACE MINERALS PLUS+®. We have a long history together, gratefully labeling their product for our professional and private clients, and now bring it to you.

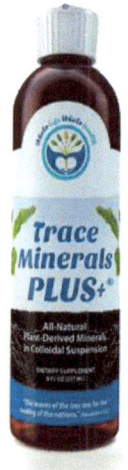

I began using the ROYAL FLUSH® many years ago, when I was on a quest for health after my appendix ruptured and nearly killed me. Even during a **40-DAY LEMONADE CLEANSE** (a liquid only fast, which you can learn more about in the book, *Your Personal Roadmap to Whole Body Cleansing*), I found the kind of *"treasures"* you see in the pictures on page 4.

Dr. Taylor and I repeated the ROYAL FLUSH® a few years ago and it took nearly six months for his stools to return to normal color and consistency.

Today we make my *"Ultimate Power Shake"* that contains ½ teaspoon of TRACE MINERALS PLUS+®, and once a week or so, we use the ROYAL FLUSH® to keep our insides squeaky clean. *Barbara Brown, MSE*

WHAT TO WATCH OUT FOR WITH LIQUID MINERALS

• How long do liquid minerals last?

This is one of our favorite questions. Think of it this way: If your liquid mineral supplement is already 60-70 million years old, how much older can it possibly get in *your* lifetime? This is *NOT* true, however, for mineral supplements, such as tablets, capsules, powders, and many other liquids, which carry expiration dates.

> **If your mineral supplement has an expiration date on it, consider a different supplement!**

• Are liquid minerals organic?

Minerals themselves are naturally organic, not to be confused with *"certified organic."* The plant-based mineral deposit that produces TRACE MINERALS PLUS+® existed well before humans farmed anything, let alone before the use of toxic chemicals associated with modern commercial farming. As much as certified organic farming helps reclaim and maintain the purity of the soil's microbiological activity, the full spectrum of minerals, which was lacking when the organic farmer began tilling the soil, is still lacking.

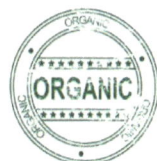

> **Farmers and home gardeners can replenish their soil's mineral-rich environment by mixing TRACE MINERALS PLUS+® directly into their soil!**

TRACE MINERALS PLUS+® was once supplied to farmers who discovered that their crops grew better, resisted disease and pests without resorting to toxic chemicals, and contained nutrients not found with other "fertilizers"!

• Are liquid minerals safe for all ages?

We can confidently testify to the safety of Trace Minerals Plus+® after well over two decades of experience in using liquid minerals and recommending them to clients with 100 percent positive results, no matter what their age or condition. Trace Minerals Plus+®, together with other responsible habits (discussed in the book *Your Personal Roadmap to Whole Body Cleansing*), helps establish and maintain an iron-clad immune system. We've discovered that no "unfriendly" organism can survive in the presence of these minerals, but they never hurt, and only support, the "friendly" organisms you need to thrive.

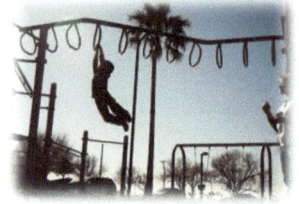

• Why would liquid minerals contain lead, arsenic and mercury?

Everyone knows that aluminum is toxic to humans, right? Yet, from 1970 and 1984, aluminum, bromine, vanadium and nickel – even arsenic and lead – were found in human milk, together with at least 56 other trace minerals, suggesting that human beings *need* minerals that were once considered toxic or of little to no benefit.

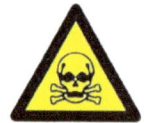

Warning Toxic

Elements like those above, and others, may be toxic in their elemental or metallic state, but when plants "digest" minerals, their electrochemical structure changes into forms that are not only nontoxic to animals and humans, but are essential to carry on activities within your body that we still don't fully understand.

God designed the natural balance between and among all the elements. We prefer to rely on His wisdom rather than that of any human, no matter how educated.

We will not endorse or recommend, much less use, supplements which a company has altered to suit its idea of what is "safe." The consequences of disturbing naturally balanced elements have often proven far worse than any supposed benefit.

OTHER IMPORTANT POINTS ABOUT LIQUID MINERALS

- ### Liquid minerals stain!

If the liquid gets on fabric, use a spot remover and wash it immediately. With some fabrics, this may not even work. It's best to keep everything away from liquid minerals except what you want them on!

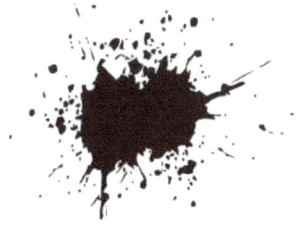

- ### Never heat liquid minerals!

Heat kills the vital properties of liquid minerals; however, a few drops in bath water can help neutralize the chlorine in tap water.

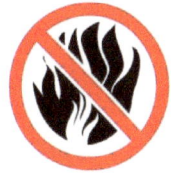

- ### Liquid minerals are highly astringent.

Never use liquid minerals directly in the eyes!

- ### Liquid minerals are super bitter!

We've never chewed on a rusty fence, but that's the image that comes to mind. You can gain first-hand experience with the bitter taste of liquid minerals by putting a drop on your tongue. YUCK!

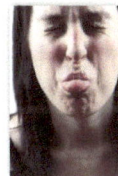

- ### Liquid minerals can sting.

When applying liquid minerals to open wounds, especially for kids and animals, mix 1 drop of minerals with 3-4 drops of water.

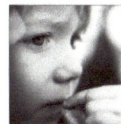

- ### No "bad guy bugs" can live with liquid minerals.

Liquid minerals naturally kill and repel unfriendly bacteria and viruses, but they'll never hurt you when used properly.

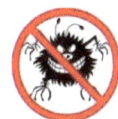

How to Get the Most from Trace Minerals Plus+®

Health and wellness are the natural consequences of taking charge and taking care of your body, mind, and spirit. Physically, your goal ought to be to cultivate an internal environment that promotes and supports your total well-being, and vigorously defends against environmental invaders.

> **Trace Minerals Plus+®**
> **helps us achieve that goal.**

Mix ¼ to ½ teaspoon into shakes, smoothies, or a glass of fresh fruit juice once a day (we find that orange and grapefruit work best). You'll be replenishing what *should* be in the food you eat but isn't, and what your body desperately needs.

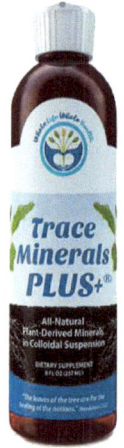

Trace Minerals Plus+® is an accurate name, because the plant deposit from which these liquid minerals are derived contains a **complete spectrum** of all known trace

> **Apart from the Royal Flush®, you may only need 1/4 to 1/2 teaspoon a day!**

and ultra-trace elements, plus minor and macro minerals. In addition, the fulvic acid in Trace Minerals Plus+® gives this solution some truly astonishing properties:

- **Energizes water** and makes it better able to carry nutrients into, and waste products away from, your cells
- **Alerts and strengthens** the immune system
- **Helps neutralize toxins**
- **Neutralizes viruses**
- **Highly absorbable** and bio-active
- Acts as a **natural antibiotic**, **antimicrobial** and **antiviral** agent

FIRST AID WITH TRACE MINERALS PLUS+®

TRACE MINERALS PLUS+® has tremendous healing properties that we have been privileged to experience firsthand, and witness in the lives of countless individuals and families over more than two decades.

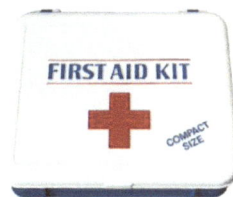

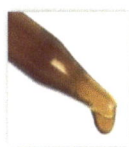

The following are some of the most common applications for which TRACE MINERALS PLUS+® have proven to deliver effective first aid.

- **Cuts**

After cleaning a wound, put a drop of TRACE MINERALS PLUS+® (or more, depending on wound size) directly on the cut or wound. This will most often cauterize the bleeding. Deeper wounds may require bandaging and pressure, but TRACE MINERALS PLUS+® will help cauterize and clean the wound until medical attention can be obtained.

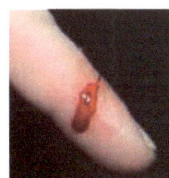

- **Burns**

Put TRACE MINERALS PLUS+® on any burn area, followed by ice. Do this twice. After the second application of minerals and ice, no blister will raise and often you won't even be able to find the burn!

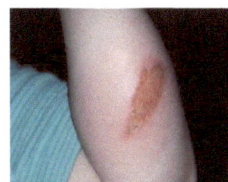

- **Sore Throats**

Put 4-5 drops of TRACE MINERALS PLUS+® in 1-2 oz. of water, gargle and swallow. Once may be enough if you catch it early. If not, repeat 3-6 times per day. The condition should clear up in 1-2 days (even Thrush and Strep Throat).

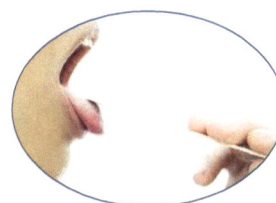

- ## Sinus Infections

Put 4-6 drops of TRACE MINERALS PLUS+® in an ounce of saline solution (salt water), with a cap that allows you to create a nasal spray. Spray and inhale the mixture through each nostril into the sinuses. Get tissues ready, because the sludge that you'll blow out is unbelievable! For impacted sinuses, more than one application may be needed, but they'll often clear within 24 hours. This method works for sinus congestion too!

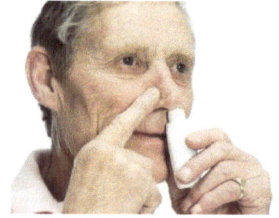

- ## Boils and Skin Eruptions

Use just like cuts and wounds. Wet a bandage pad with 2-3 drops of TRACE MINERALS PLUS+® and cover the area. Do this twice a day for as long as needed. Boils usually clear up in a few days.

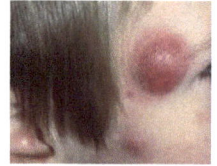

- ## Tooth Abscesses (or impacted teeth)

Soak a Q-Tip™ with 3-4 drops of TRACE MINERALS PLUS+® and rub into the gum line at the involved tooth *(Note: You will taste the minerals)*. Repeat this a few times a day until you can get to your dentist, or until the abscess clears or resolves itself; but don't wait more than a couple of days.

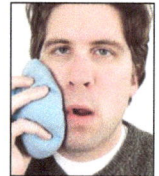

- **Additional Help:** After applying TRACE MINERALS PLUS+®, open a capsule of probiotics and massage into the gum line.

- ## Cold and Chancre Sores

Apply 1 drop of TRACE MINERALS PLUS+® directly to the area. Use a Q-Tip™ if you like. Liquid minerals will stain external sores, but they can clear up in less than 24 hours. For internal sores, use as described for tooth remedies above and repeat as needed.

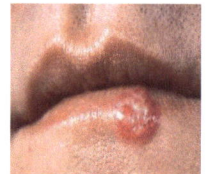

• Internal Bleeding

Mix 1 teaspoon of TRACE MINERALS PLUS+® in orange or grapefruit juice, and drink daily for 3 days. If the stool turns black, continue for 21 days. Stool should change to brown within that time. If not, seek medical help.

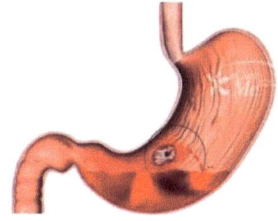

• Sunburn

Apply TRACE MINERALS PLUS+® directly to the sunburned area (use a soaked cotton pad). If the area is quite large, put 1 tablespoon of TRACE MINERALS PLUS+® in a tub of water that is just warm enough to get in, and bathe for 10-20 minutes. You may need to repeat this daily until the burn heals, depending on its severity.

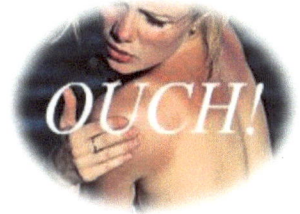

• Hemorrhoids

If hemorrhoids aren't bleeding, put 3-4 drops of TRACE MINERALS PLUS+® on a single square of toilet paper folded in quarters. Apply the minerals directly on the hemorrhoids with pressure; then apply ointment over the area (our favorite is "Neem" ointment). For bleeding hemorrhoids, make a "sitz bath" of warm water and a teaspoon of TRACE MINERALS PLUS+®. Sit in the solution for at least 5 minutes and repeat twice daily until tissues heal enough to use the procedure above, (usually 1-2 days).

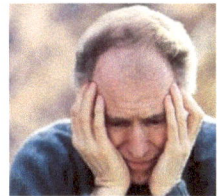

• Systemic Yeast Infections (Candida)

Use ¼ teaspoon of TRACE MINERALS PLUS+® 3 times per day in water (remember, this tastes bitter). Avoid *ALL* dairy, grains, refined sugar, and fruit. This can take several weeks to clear up.

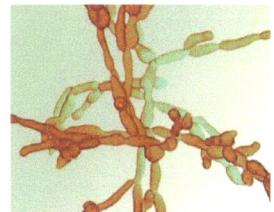

- ## Vaginal Yeast and Vaginitis

Prepare a douche container filled with sterile saline. Add 4 drops of TRACE MINERALS PLUS+® and apply 1-2 times per day. This will often clear up even the most raging infections in 1-3 days.

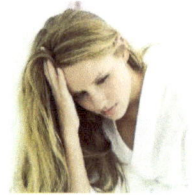

- ## Ear Infections

Put 1-2 drops of TRACE MINERALS PLUS+® directly into the affected ear, pack gently with cotton, and apply moist heat (hot water bottles work well), while lying on the affected side. Repeat 2-3 times a day. Infections often clear in a day or less.

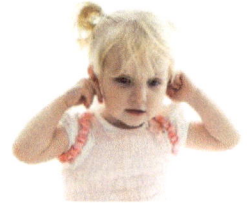

- ## Traveling

Take *at least* a teaspoon of TRACE MINERALS PLUS+® per day when traveling to avoid diarrhea from unfamiliar water and foods.

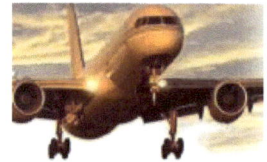

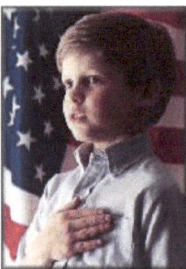

HERE'S OUR PLEDGE: **We will *ONLY* share what passes our "100% test." Any time something creates more stress than benefit, we won't waste your time.**

"...let your word be 'Yes, Yes,' or 'No, No.'" (Matthew 5:37)

27

Tons More "How To's" and Other Treasures
at CLEANSINGROADMAP.com

➢ **VIDEOS** – Access 20 videos answering the most important questions about Nutritional Cleansing and bonus videos which ensure your success. We've done the work. Just watch and follow along!

➢ **ACTION GUIDES** – Let us walk you through the steps that lead to success, whether it's losing weight, getting through caffeine withdrawal, or getting the most from your cleanses!

➢ **RESOURCES AND BEST SOURCES** – Find out what's worth watching and who's worth tracking! If you want to take your precious time searching through mountains of information and countless web sites for the stuff you need and the information you seek, be our guest, but chances are, we've already found it!

➢ **THE ESSENTIAL NON-NEGOTIABLE FIVE** – Discover the answer to the most frequently asked question we hear: "What do YOU take every day to stay young and healthy?"

➢ **RECOMMENDED READING** – When it comes to health and wellness, authorities abound and very few agree. The good news is that the list is fairly short of the authors we trust, and they get results. Have an authority you'd like us to check out? Let us know. We'll tell you what we think!

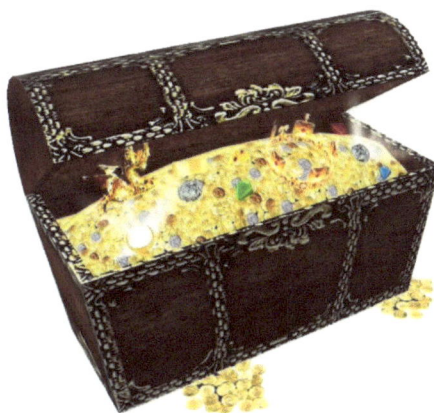

Go to CLEANSINGROADMAP.com

> *"First clean the inside of the cup, so that the outside may be clean too."* (Matthew 23:26)

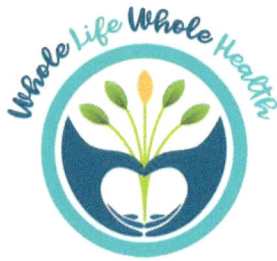

Divine Health
is Your Original Design

www.ingramcontent.com/pod-product-compliance
Lightning Source LLC
Chambersburg PA
CBHW060829270326
41931CB00003B/110